KIDNEY DISEASE DIET COOKBOOK FOR WOMEN

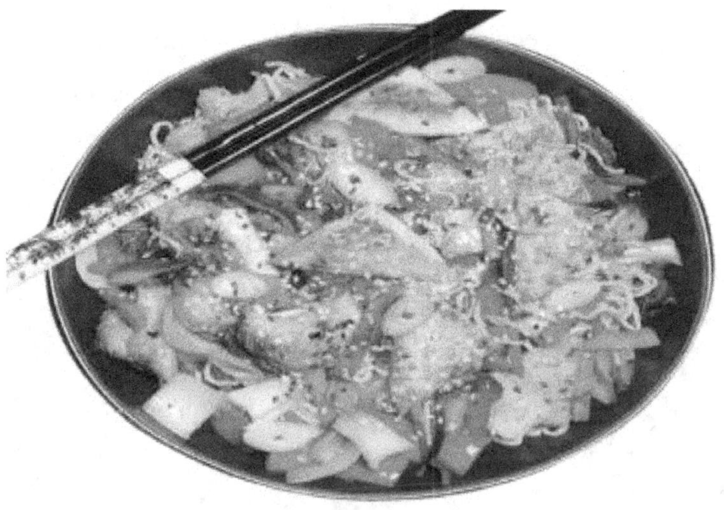

The Ultimate Guide To Manage Chronic Kidney Disease And Improve Renal Function In Women With Healthy And Delicious Low Sodium, Potassium And Phosphorus Recipes

Katherine J. Filer

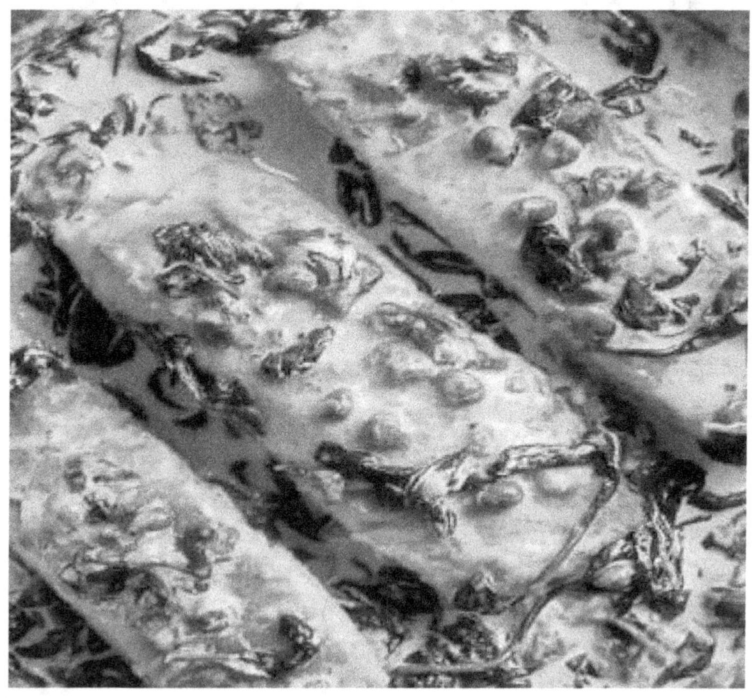

Table of Contents

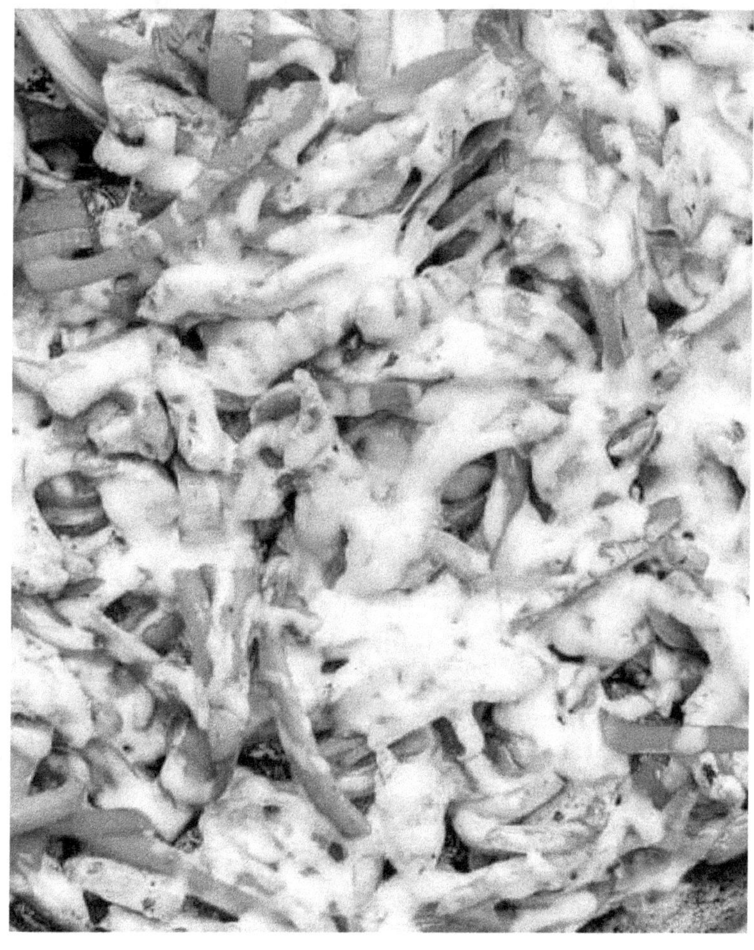

INTRODUCTION

Welcome to "Kidney disease diet cookbook for women," a culinary journey dedicated to empowering women battling kidney disease through the healing power of food. This cookbook is more than just a collection of recipes; it's a testament to the strength and resilience of women who face kidney disease every day. My inspiration to create this book stemmed from a personal story, my mother's brave fight against kidney disease. Watching her struggle and triumph inspired me to explore how diet could become her strongest ally.

Kidney disease often lurks silently, disproportionately affecting women worldwide. It's a battle fought on many fronts, and diet is a crucial weapon. This cookbook serves as your guide, offering not just recipes, but a new perspective on food as a source of healing and joy. Every dish in this book is tailored to meet the nutritional needs of women with kidney disease, emphasizing ingredients that support kidney health.

What sets "Kidney disease diet cookbook for women "apart is its dedication to simplicity and flavor. Whether you're a novice in the kitchen or a seasoned cook, these recipes are designed to be accessible, easy to prepare, and delicious. From hearty breakfasts to nourishing dinners, each recipe is a celebration of flavor that respects dietary restrictions without compromising taste.

I've included stories from women who have transformed their health through diet, alongside their favorite recipes from this book. Their journeys are as diverse as the recipes themselves, yet they share a common thread - the transformative power of mindful eating.

As you turn these pages, you'll find a range of recipes, practical meal plans, and nutritional insights. But more importantly, you'll find hope and empowerment. This book is not just about managing kidney disease; it's about thriving despite it.

Join me on this delicious journey to better health. Let each recipe be a step towards empowerment, a celebration of your health, and a tribute to the resilience that defines us as women. Welcome to "Kidney disease diet cookbook for women."

CHAPTER 1

Understanding Kidney Disease

Kidney disease, a significant health concern worldwide, refers to the gradual loss of kidney function over time. The kidneys, a pair of bean-shaped organs located at the back of the abdomen, play a crucial role in maintaining overall health. Their primary function is to filter waste products and excess fluids from the blood, which are then excreted in the urine. When the kidneys are damaged, they cannot perform this vital function effectively, leading to the accumulation of harmful substances in the body.

Types of Kidney Disease

1. Chronic Kidney Disease (CKD): CKD is a long-term condition where the kidneys progressively lose their function. It's often a result of conditions that put a strain on the kidneys, like high blood pressure and diabetes.

2. Acute Kidney Injury (AKI): AKI is an acute phase of renal injury or failure that occurs in a matter of hours or days. AKI makes it difficult for your kidneys to maintain the proper balance of fluid in your body and leads to the accumulation of waste products in your blood.

3. Polycystic Kidney Disease (PKD): This is a genetic disorder characterized by the growth of numerous cysts in the kidneys, which can interfere with their normal function.

4. Glomerulonephritis: This refers to a range of conditions that cause inflammation of the kidneys' tiny filters, or glomeruli. It can be acute or chronic and can lead to CKD if not managed properly.

5. Kidney Stones: While not a direct form of kidney disease, kidney stones can lead to kidney damage if they cause persistent obstruction or infection.

Causes Of Kidney Disease

- Diabetes: High blood sugar levels, a result of diabetes, can damage the blood vessels in the kidneys.

- High Blood Pressure (Hypertension): High blood pressure can damage the tiny blood vessels in the kidneys.

- Autoimmune Diseases: Conditions like lupus can cause the immune system to attack the kidneys.

- Genetic Disorders: Such as PKD.

- Prolonged Urinary Tract Obstructions: Due to conditions like kidney stones, enlarged prostate, and some cancers.

- Recurrent Kidney Infection: Also known as pyelonephritis.

Symptoms of Kidney Disease

In the early stages, kidney disease often has no symptoms and can go unnoticed until it is advanced. However, as the disease progresses, symptoms may include:

- Fatigue and weakness
- Swelling in the feet and ankles
- Increased or decreased urination
- Shortness of breath
- Persistent nausea
- Blood in the urine
- Elevated blood pressure
- Decreased mental sharpness

Preventive Measures

Preventing kidney disease involves managing its risk factors and leading a kidney-friendly lifestyle:

1. **Control Blood Sugar:** For those with diabetes, effective management of blood sugar levels is crucial. Regular monitoring and adherence to a diabetes care plan can prevent or delay the onset of kidney damage.

2. **Maintain Healthy Blood Pressure:** High blood pressure is a significant risk factor for kidney disease. Controlling

blood pressure through diet, exercise, and medication (if prescribed) can reduce the risk.

3. Healthy Lifestyle Choices: This includes maintaining a healthy weight, exercising regularly, and eating a balanced diet low in sodium and processed foods.

4. Avoid Smoking and Excessive Alcohol Consumption: Smoking can damage blood vessels, reducing blood flow to the kidneys, while excessive alcohol can cause variations in the blood flow to the kidneys, impacting their function.

5. Stay Hydrated: Adequate water intake helps the kidneys clear sodium and toxins from the body.

6. Regular Screening: If you have risk factors for kidney disease, regular kidney function screening is essential. This can help detect kidney damage early and prevent progression.

7. Medication Management: Some medications, especially over-the-counter pain relievers, can harm the kidneys if taken regularly over a long period. It's crucial to discuss medication use with a healthcare provider.

Foods To Eat And Avoid

A kidney disease diet focuses on managing the intake of certain nutrients to prevent further damage to the kidneys. This diet varies depending on the stage of kidney disease, but some general guidelines apply. It's important to work with a healthcare provider or a dietitian for personalized advice. Here's a general overview of foods to eat and avoid for optimum kidney health:

Foods to Eat

1. Fruits and Vegetables: Fresh fruits and vegetables are generally good for kidney health. They are high in vitamins, minerals, and fiber while being low in sodium and phosphorus. Recommended options include red bell peppers, cabbage, cauliflower, garlic, onions, apples, cranberries, blueberries, and raspberries.

2. Whole Grains: Whole grains are a healthier choice than refined grains because they contain more fiber and nutrients. Options include barley, buckwheat, bulgur, whole wheat, and oats.

3. Lean Proteins: High-quality protein is important, but it should be consumed in moderation. Good sources are chicken, fish, egg whites, and plant-based proteins like lentils, chickpeas, and kidney beans.

4. Heart-Healthy Fats: Unsaturated fats are beneficial for overall health and can be found in foods like olive oil, avocado, nuts, and seeds.

5. Low-Phosphorus Dairy Alternatives: For those who need to limit phosphorus, almond milk or rice milk can be good alternatives to regular milk.

6. Low-Sodium Options: Fresh or frozen unsalted ingredients are preferable to canned or processed foods.

Foods to Avoid or Limit

1. High-Sodium Foods: Salt can cause fluid retention and increase blood pressure, stressing the kidneys. Avoid processed foods, canned soups, packaged snacks, and condiments like soy sauce.

2. High-Potassium Foods: Depending on individual restrictions, high-potassium foods might need to be limited. These include bananas, oranges, potatoes, spinach, and tomatoes.

3. High-Phosphorus Foods: Phosphorus can build up in the blood when kidneys are not functioning properly. Foods rich in phosphorus like dairy products, nuts, seeds, and whole grains may need to be limited.

4. Processed Meats: These are high in sodium and phosphorus. Examples include deli meats, sausages, and canned meats.

5. Alcohol: It can stress the kidneys and affect the body's ability to regulate fluids and electrolytes.

6. Sugary Foods: Excessive sugar can lead to weight gain, high blood pressure, and diabetes, all of which can strain the kidneys.

Core Benefits Of Following A Kidney Disease Diet Cookbook For Women

1. Slows the Progression of Kidney Disease: Adhering to a kidney-friendly diet can help slow down the progression of kidney disease. By controlling intake of nutrients like sodium, potassium, and phosphorus, which kidneys struggle to filter in later stages of disease, the diet eases the kidneys' workload.

2. Maintains Optimal Blood Pressure Levels: High blood pressure is a common cause and consequence of kidney disease. A kidney disease diet, low in sodium and saturated fats, helps in managing blood pressure levels, thus reducing the risk of further kidney damage.

3. Regulates Blood Sugar Levels: For women with diabetes, a leading cause of kidney disease, this diet aids in controlling blood sugar levels. By incorporating low glycemic index foods and controlling carbohydrate intake, the diet helps in managing diabetes effectively.

4. Prevents Accumulation of Harmful Substances: Impaired kidneys may not effectively filter waste products. A kidney disease diet limits foods that produce high levels of waste products, thereby preventing harmful accumulation in the blood.

5. Manages Weight: Obesity can be a risk factor for kidney disease. A kidney-friendly diet often aligns with principles of healthy eating and weight management, thus helping women maintain a healthy weight.

6. Improves Energy Levels and Overall Well-being: By ensuring a balanced intake of all essential nutrients, the diet can enhance overall health, leading to improved energy levels and wellbeing.

7. Reduces the Risk of Kidney Stones: Certain types of kidney stones are related to dietary factors. A kidney disease diet, by controlling intake of stone-forming nutrients like oxalates and calcium, can help in preventing the formation of new kidney stones.

8. Addresses Unique Nutritional Needs of Women: Women have specific nutritional needs, especially during phases like menstruation, pregnancy, and menopause. A kidney disease diet tailored for women takes these unique requirements into account, ensuring optimal health.

9. Enhances Heart Health: There's a strong link between kidney and cardiovascular health. A kidney disease diet that's low in sodium and unhealthy fats contributes to better heart health, reducing the risk of heart diseases, which are more prevalent in women as they age.

10. Empowers Self-Care and Health Awareness: Following this diet encourages women to take an active role in their health management, promoting greater awareness of food choices and their impact on overall health.

List Of 20 Healthy Shopping Ingredients

1. White Rice: Lower in potassium than brown rice, it's a good carbohydrate source.

2. Bell Peppers: High in vitamins A and C, bell peppers add flavor without unwanted potassium.

3. Cabbage: Low in potassium, rich in vitamins K and C, and versatile for salads and cooking.

4. Cauliflower: A low-potassium alternative to high-potassium vegetables, great for mashing or roasting.

5. Garlic and Onions: Flavorful additions to dishes without the need for salt.

6. Berries (Blueberries, Strawberries): Low in potassium, high in antioxidants and vitamins.

7. Apples and Pears: Fruits with lower potassium levels, perfect for snacking.

8. Egg Whites: High-quality protein source without the phosphorus found in yolks.

9. Chicken Breast: Lean protein, opt for fresh rather than processed to avoid added sodium.

10. Olive Oil: Healthy fat for cooking and dressings.

11. White Bread or Low-Sodium Bread: Lower in potassium and phosphorus than whole wheat varieties.

12. Rice Milk or Almond Milk (Unenriched): Non-dairy alternatives low in potassium and phosphorus.

13. Green Beans: Low-potassium vegetable, can be steamed, boiled, or stir-fried.

14. Fresh or Frozen Fish (like Cod, Tilapia): Good protein source, opt for fresh or frozen without added sodium.

15. Egg Noodles or Refined Pasta: Better options than whole grain versions for lower phosphorus.

16. Low-Sodium Broth: For soups and cooking, a better choice than regular broths high in sodium.

17. Herbs and Spices (except high-potassium herbs like potassium chloride): For flavoring food without salt.

18. Unsalted Butter or Margarine: Use in moderation for cooking and flavor.

19. Honey or White Sugar: As sweeteners, but use in moderation for overall health.

20. Water and Clear Beverages: Such as lemonade or homemade iced tea without added sugars.

Shopping Tips:

- Always read labels for sodium, potassium, and phosphorus content.
- Choose fresh or frozen produce over canned, or select canned items labeled "no salt added" or "low sodium".
- Avoid processed foods and deli meats which are typically high in sodium.
- Be cautious with dairy products, as they are high in phosphorus. Limit to small portions.

Complications Of Kidney Disease If The Right Diet Isn't Adopted

1. Fluid Retention: Without dietary management, excess fluid can build up, leading to swelling in the legs, ankles, and feet, high blood pressure, and pulmonary edema (fluid in the lungs).

2. Electrolyte Imbalances: Kidneys help balance electrolytes like potassium, sodium, and phosphorus. An improper diet can lead to imbalances, causing conditions like hyperkalemia (high potassium) which can affect heart rhythm and increase the risk of a heart attack.

3. Bone and Mineral Disorders: Advanced kidney disease can disrupt the balance of minerals in the body, leading to weakened bones, increased risk of bone fractures, and vascular calcification, which can contribute to heart disease.

4. Anemia: Kidneys produce the hormone erythropoietin, which stimulates red blood cell production. Kidney disease can lower this hormone's levels, causing anemia, which leads to fatigue and weakness.

5. Malnutrition: Inadequate nutrition can result from dietary restrictions and changes in metabolism due to kidney disease, leading to malnutrition and muscle wasting.

6. Acidosis: The kidneys help regulate the body's acid-base balance. Failure to manage diet can lead to metabolic acidosis, a condition where the body accumulates too much acid or cannot remove enough acid, causing muscle deterioration and affecting heart and lung function.

7. Heart and Vascular Disease: Kidney disease increases the risk of cardiovascular diseases. A poor diet, especially one high in sodium and unhealthy fats, can exacerbate this risk, leading to conditions like hypertension, heart disease, and stroke.

8. Uremia: If kidneys can't filter waste products from the blood, it can lead to uremia, characterized by symptoms like nausea, fatigue, itching, difficulty concentrating, and loss of appetite.

9. Potassium Overload: High potassium levels can lead to dangerous heart rhythm disturbances and even cardiac arrest.

10. Phosphorus Accumulation: Excess phosphorus can leach calcium from the bones, weakening them, and deposit in blood vessels, muscles, and other organs, impairing their function.

How to follow a kidney disease diet

1. Understand Your Individual Dietary Needs: Kidney disease varies in severity, and dietary needs can differ based on individual health factors and the stage of kidney disease. Consult with a healthcare provider or dietitian for personalized advice.

2. Reduce Sodium Intake: Excessive salt intake can lead to fluid retention and raise blood pressure, worsening kidney function. Opt for fresh foods over processed ones, avoid adding salt during cooking or at the table, and be cautious with high-sodium condiments.

3. Control Protein Consumption: Protein is essential but in controlled amounts. In kidney disease, consuming too much protein can put a strain on the kidneys. Lean meats, poultry, fish, and plant-based proteins are good choices.

4. Monitor Potassium Levels: Potassium is a mineral crucial for heart function, but too much can be harmful in kidney disease. Depending on your kidney function, you may need to limit high-potassium foods like bananas, oranges, potatoes, and tomatoes.

5. Manage Phosphorus Intake: High phosphorus levels can lead to bone and heart problems. Avoid or limit foods high in phosphorus such as dairy products, nuts, seeds, beans, and whole grains.

6. Choose the Right Carbohydrates: Focus on complex carbohydrates like vegetables, fruits, and whole grains. Avoid simple sugars and sweets as they can cause spikes in blood sugar levels.

7. Stay Hydrated: Proper hydration is important, but too much fluid can lead to complications. Your fluid intake might need to be adjusted based on your stage of kidney disease.

8. Limit Alcohol and Avoid Smoking: Alcohol can affect the ability of your kidneys to function and smoking can worsen kidney disease.

9. Read Food Labels: Become vigilant about reading food labels to check for sodium, potassium, and phosphorus content, especially in processed and packaged foods.

10. Prepare Food Healthily: Use cooking methods that require less salt and fat, such as steaming, grilling, or baking. Flavor foods with herbs and spices instead of salt.

11. Regular Monitoring: Regularly check in with your healthcare provider to monitor your kidney function and adjust your diet as needed.

12. Stay Informed: Keep yourself educated about kidney disease and nutrition. Attend workshops, join support groups, or follow reliable online resources.

13. Meal Planning: Plan your meals ahead to ensure you stick to your kidney-friendly diet. Preparing meals at home gives you better control over ingredients.

14. Balance Your Diet: Ensure your diet is balanced with the right mix of proteins, carbohydrates, fats, vitamins, and minerals.

15. Take Prescribed Supplements: If recommended by your healthcare provider, take vitamin and mineral supplements to compensate for the dietary restrictions.

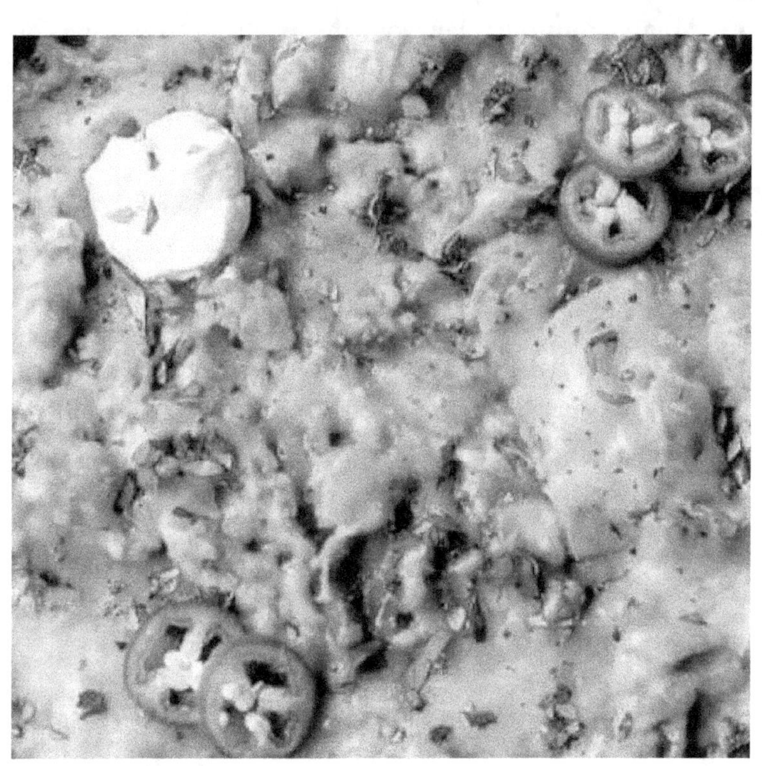

CHAPTER 2

BREAKFAST RECIPES

1. Creamy Oatmeal with Berries

Prep Time: 5 minutes

Cooking Time: 15 minutes

Serving Size: 1

Ingredients:

- 1/2 cup rolled oats

- 1 cup low-fat milk

- 1/4 cup fresh mixed berries (blueberries, strawberries, raspberries)

- 1 tablespoon honey

- 1/4 teaspoon cinnamon

- 1/4 teaspoon vanilla extract

Instructions:

1. In a saucepan, combine rolled oats and milk. Cook over medium heat, stirring occasionally, until the oatmeal thickens (about 10-15 minutes).

2. Remove from heat and stir in honey, cinnamon, and vanilla extract.

3. Top with fresh mixed berries.

Nutritional Information (per serving):

- Calories: 250

- Protein: 8g

- Sodium: 100mg

- Potassium: 220mg

- Phosphorus: 150ml

2. Scrambled Egg Whites with Spinach

Prep Time: 5 minutes

Cooking Time: 10 minutes

Serving Size: 1

Ingredients:

- 3 egg whites

- 1/2 cup fresh spinach, chopped

- 1/4 cup low-fat feta cheese

- Pepper and salt

Instructions:

1. In a bowl, whisk the egg whites until frothy.

2. Heat a non-stick skillet over medium heat, add the chopped spinach, and sauté until wilted.

3. Pour the egg whites over the spinach, add feta cheese, and scramble until cooked through.

4. Season with pepper and salt.

Nutritional Information (per serving):

- Calories: 180

- Protein: 25g

- Sodium: 420mg

- Potassium: 260mg

- Phosphorus: 160mg

3. Banana Almond Smoothie

Prep Time: 5 minutes

Serving Size: 1

Ingredients:

- 1 ripe banana

- 1 cup unsweetened almond milk

- 1 tablespoon almond butter

- 1/2 teaspoon honey (optional)

- Ice cubes (optional)

Instructions:

1. Blend the banana, almond milk, almond butter, and honey until smooth.

2. Add ice cubes and blend again for a colder, thicker consistency.

Nutritional Information (per serving):

- Calories: 210

- Protein: 4g

- Sodium: 150mg

- Potassium: 380mg

- Phosphorus: 90mg

4. Greek Yogurt Parfait with Nuts and Berries

Prep Time: 5 minutes

Serving Size: 1

Ingredients:

- 1/2 cup low-fat Greek yogurt

- 1/4 cup mixed nuts (almonds, walnuts)

- 1/4 cup fresh mixed berries

- 1 teaspoon honey

Instructions:

1. In a glass or bowl, layer Greek yogurt, mixed nuts, and fresh mixed berries.

2. Drizzle honey on top.

Nutritional Information (per serving):

- Calories: 320

- Protein: 14g

- Sodium: 60mg

- Potassium: 200mg

- Phosphorus: 120mg

5. Spinach and Mushroom Breakfast Quesadilla

Prep Time: 10 minutes

Cooking Time: 10 minutes

Serving Size: 1

Ingredients:

- 1 whole wheat tortilla

- 1/2 cup fresh spinach, chopped

- 1/4 cup sliced mushrooms

- 2 egg whites

- 1/4 cup low-fat shredded mozzarella cheese

- Pepper and salt

Instructions:

1. In a non-stick skillet, sauté chopped spinach and sliced mushrooms until tender. Remove from the skillet and set aside.

2. In the same skillet, cook the egg whites until set.

3. Place the whole wheat tortilla in the skillet, then layer with sautéed vegetables, scrambled egg whites, and mozzarella cheese.

4. Fold the tortilla in half and cook until the cheese melts and the tortilla is golden brown.

5. Season with pepper and salt.

Nutritional Information (per serving):

- Calories: 320

- Protein: 24g

- Sodium: 400mg

- Potassium: 380mg

- Phosphorus: 170mg

6. Quinoa Breakfast Bowl

Prep Time: 10 minutes

Cooking Time: 15 minutes

Serving Size: 1

Ingredients:

- 1/2 cup cooked quinoa

- 1/4 cup low-fat Greek yogurt

- 1/4 cup diced fresh mango

- 1 tablespoon chopped almonds

- 1/2 teaspoon honey (optional)

Instructions:

1. In a bowl, layer cooked quinoa, Greek yogurt, diced mango, and chopped almonds.

2. Drizzle with honey if desired.

Nutritional Information (per serving):

- Calories: 280

- Protein: 13g

- Sodium: 40mg

- Potassium: 250mg

- Phosphorus: 150mg

7. Sweet Potato Hash with Eggs

Prep Time: 15 minutes

Cooking Time: 20 minutes

Serving Size: 1

Ingredients:

- 1 small sweet potato, diced

- 1/4 cup diced red bell pepper

- 1/4 cup diced onion

- 2 eggs

- 1 tablespoon olive oil

- Pepper and salt

Instructions:

1. Heat olive oil in a skillet over medium heat. Add diced sweet potato, red bell pepper, and onion. Sauté until sweet potatoes are tender and slightly crispy (about 15 minutes).

2. Create two small wells in the sweet potato hash and crack eggs into them. Cover and cook until the egg whites are set but the yolks are still runny (or to your desired doneness).

3. Season with pepper and salt.

Nutritional Information (per serving):

- Calories: 330

- Protein: 11g

- Sodium: 140mg

- Potassium: 430mg

- Phosphorus: 130mg

8. Blueberry Cottage Cheese Pancakes

Prep Time: 10 minutes

Cooking Time: 10 minutes

Serving Size: 2 pancakes

Ingredients:

- 1/2 cup low-fat cottage cheese

- 2 eggs

- 1/4 cup whole wheat flour

- 1/4 cup fresh blueberries

- 1/2 teaspoon vanilla extract

- 1/4 teaspoon baking powder

- Cooking spray

Instructions:

1. In a blender, combine cottage cheese, eggs, whole wheat flour, vanilla extract, and baking powder. Blend until smooth.

2. Gently fold in fresh blueberries.

3. Heat a non-stick skillet over medium heat and lightly coat with cooking spray. Pour small portions of the batter to make pancakes.

4. Cook until surface bubbles appear, then turn and continue cooking until golden brown.

Nutritional Information (per serving - 2 pancakes):

- Calories: 260

- Protein: 22g

- Sodium: 280mg

- Potassium: 220mg

- Phosphorus: 150mg

9. Avocado and Tomato Toast

Prep Time: 5 minutes

Serving Size: 1

Ingredients:

- 1 slice whole grain bread, toasted

- 1/2 ripe avocado, mashed

- 1/2 small tomato, sliced

- 1 teaspoon lemon juice

- Pepper and salt

Instructions:

1. Spread mashed avocado on the toasted bread.

2. Top with sliced tomatoes, drizzle with lemon juice, and season with pepper and salt.

Nutritional Information (per serving):

- Calories: 180

- Protein: 4g

- Sodium: 170mg

- Potassium: 370mg

- Phosphorus: 100mg

10. Chia Seed Pudding

Prep Time: 5 minutes (plus chilling time)

Serving Size: 1

Ingredients:

- 2 tablespoons chia seeds

- 1/2 cup unsweetened almond milk

- 1/4 cup diced fresh pineapple

- 1/4 teaspoon vanilla extract

- 1/2 teaspoon honey (optional)

Instructions:

1. In a jar, combine chia seeds, almond milk, vanilla extract, and diced pineapple. Stir well.

2. Cover and refrigerate for at least 2 hours or overnight until it thickens.

3. Drizzle with honey if desired before serving.

Nutritional Information (per serving):

- Calories: 180

- Protein: 4g

- Sodium: 80mg

- Potassium: 160mg

- Phosphorus: 90mg

LUNCH RECIPES

1. Creamy Chicken and Vegetable Soup

- **Prep Time:** 15 minutes

- **Cooking Time:** 30 minutes

- **Serving Size:** 1

Ingredients:

- 150g boneless, skinless chicken breast, diced

- 1/2 cup diced carrots

- 1/2 cup diced celery

- 1/4 cup chopped onion

- 1 garlic clove, minced

- 1 cup low-sodium chicken broth

- 1/2 cup low-fat milk

- 1 tsp olive oil

- Pepper and salt

Instructions:

1. In a pot, heat olive oil over medium heat. Add garlic and onion, sauté until translucent.

2. Cook the chicken until it loses its pink color.

3. Stir in carrots and celery, cook for 5 minutes.

4. Pour in chicken broth and bring to a boil. Simmer for 15 minutes.

5. Add milk, salt, and pepper, and simmer for an additional 5 minutes.

Nutritional Information (per serving):

- Calories: 280

- Protein: 25g

- Sodium: 280mg

- Potassium: 450mg

- Phosphorus: 200mg

2. Lemon Garlic Shrimp and Asparagus

- **Prep Time:** 10 minutes

- **Cooking Time:** 15 minutes

- **Serving Size:** 1

Ingredients:

- 150g large shrimp, peeled and deveined

- 1/2 cup asparagus spears, trimmed and cut into 2-inch pieces

- 1 garlic clove, minced

- 1 tsp olive oil

- Juice of half a lemon

- Pepper and salt

Instructions:

1. Warm up the olive oil in a skillet over a medium heat. Add garlic and sauté for 1 minute.

2. Add shrimp and cook until they turn pink, about 3-4 minutes.

3. Add asparagus, lemon juice, salt, and pepper. Cook for an additional 5-7 minutes, until asparagus is tender.

Nutritional Information (per serving):

- Calories: 180

- Protein: 25g

- Sodium: 200mg

- Potassium: 400mg

- Phosphorus: 180mg

3. Quinoa and Vegetable Stir-Fry

- **Prep Time:** 15 minutes

- **Cooking Time:** 20 minutes

- **Serving Size:** 1

Ingredients:

- 1/2 cup cooked quinoa

- 1/2 cup mixed vegetables (bell peppers, broccoli, snap peas)

- 1/4 cup diced tofu

- 1 garlic clove, minced

- 1 tsp low-sodium soy sauce

- 1 tsp olive oil

- Pepper and salt

Instructions:

1. Warm up the olive oil in a pan over a medium heat. Add garlic and tofu, cook until tofu is lightly browned.

2. Add mixed vegetables and stir-fry for 5-7 minutes.

3. Add cooked quinoa, soy sauce, salt, and pepper. Stir well and cook for an additional 2-3 minutes.

Nutritional Information (per serving):

- Calories: 300

- Protein: 15g

- Sodium: 220mg

- Potassium: 250mg

- Phosphorus: 150mg

4. Salmon and Spinach Salad

- **Prep Time:** 10 minutes

- **Cooking Time:** 15 minutes

- **Serving Size:** 1

Ingredients:

- 150g salmon fillet

- 2 cups fresh spinach leaves

- 1/4 cup cherry tomatoes, halved

- 1/4 cup cucumber slices

- 1 tbsp balsamic vinaigrette dressing

- 1 tsp olive oil

- Pepper and salt

Instructions:

1. Season salmon with pepper and salt. Heat olive oil in a pan over medium-high heat. Cook salmon for 3-4 minutes per side until it flakes easily.

2. In a bowl, combine spinach, cherry tomatoes, and cucumber.

3. Drizzle with balsamic vinaigrette dressing and top with cooked salmon.

Nutritional Information (per serving):

- Calories: 320

- Protein: 30g

- Sodium: 220mg

- Potassium: 600mg

- Phosphorus: 250mg

5. Mushroom and Spinach Omelette

- **Prep Time:** 10 minutes

- **Cooking Time:** 10 minutes

- **Serving Size:** 1

Ingredients:

- 2 large eggs

- 1/2 cup sliced mushrooms

- 1 cup fresh spinach leaves

- 1/4 cup diced onion

- 1 tsp olive oil

- Pepper and salt

Instructions:

1. In a non-stick skillet, heat olive oil over medium heat. Add mushrooms and onions, sauté until softened.

2. Whisk eggs in a bowl and pour over the mushrooms and onions. Cook until set.

3. Add fresh spinach leaves on one side of the omelette, fold the other side over it.

4. Cook for an additional minute, then serve.

Nutritional Information (per serving):

- Calories: 250

- Protein: 17g

- Sodium: 200mg

- Potassium: 450mg

- Phosphorus: 220mg

6. Grilled Lemon Herb Chicken Salad

- **Prep Time:** 15 minutes

- **Cooking Time:** 15 minutes

- **Serving Size:** 1

Ingredients:

- 150g boneless, skinless chicken breast

- 2 cups mixed greens (lettuce, spinach, arugula)

- 1/4 cup cherry tomatoes, halved

- 1/4 cup cucumber slices

- 1 tbsp lemon juice

- 1 tsp olive oil

- Fresh herbs (such as basil or parsley) for garnish

- Salt and pepper to taste

Instructions:

1. Season chicken with salt, pepper, and lemon juice. Grill until cooked through.

2. Slice grilled chicken and set aside.

3. In a bowl, combine mixed greens, cherry tomatoes, and cucumber.

4. Drizzle with olive oil, add grilled chicken slices, and garnish with fresh herbs.

Nutritional Information (per serving):

- Calories: 280

- Protein: 30g

- Sodium: 200mg

- Potassium: 400mg

- Phosphorus: 180mg

7. Black Bean and Vegetable Tacos

- **Prep Time:** 15 minutes

- **Cooking Time:** 15 minutes

- **Serving Size:** 2 tacos

Ingredients:

- 1/2 cup canned black beans, drained and rinsed

- 1/2 cup diced bell peppers (mixed colors)

- 1/4 cup diced red onion

- 1/4 cup chopped fresh cilantro

- 2 whole-grain tortillas

- 2 tbsp low-fat sour cream (optional)

- 1 tsp olive oil

- Salt and pepper to taste

Instructions:

1. Heat olive oil in a skillet over medium heat. Add diced peppers and onions, sauté until softened.

2. Add black beans, salt, and pepper, and cook for an additional 3-4 minutes.

3. Warm the whole-grain tortillas in the skillet.

4. Fill each tortilla with the black bean and vegetable mixture, and top with fresh cilantro. Add a dollop of low-fat sour cream if desired.

Nutritional Information (per serving - 2 tacos):

- Calories: 320

- Protein: 10g

- Sodium: 220mg

- Potassium: 300mg

- Phosphorus: 130mg

8. Baked Lemon Garlic Tilapia

- **Prep Time:** 10 minutes

- **Cooking Time:** 20 minutes

- **Serving Size:** 1

Ingredients:

- 150g tilapia fillet

- 1 clove garlic, minced

- 1/2 lemon, sliced

- 1 tsp olive oil

- Salt and pepper to taste

- Fresh parsley for garnish

Instructions:

1. Preheat the oven to 375°F (190°C).

2. Place tilapia fillet on a baking sheet lined with parchment paper.

3. Rub with olive oil, minced garlic, salt, and pepper.

4. Top with lemon slices and bake for 15-20 minutes until the fish flakes easily.

5. Garnish with fresh parsley before serving.

Nutritional Information (per serving):

- Calories: 180

- Protein: 30g

- Sodium: 100mg

- Potassium: 300mg

- Phosphorus: 180mg

9. Vegetable and Lentil Soup

- **Prep Time:** 15 minutes

- **Cooking Time:** 35 minutes

- **Serving Size:** 1

Ingredients:

- 1/2 cup dried green or brown lentils, rinsed

- 1/2 cup diced carrots

- 1/2 cup diced celery

- 1/4 cup diced onion

- 1 garlic clove, minced

- 4 cups low-sodium vegetable broth

- 1 tsp olive oil

- 1/2 tsp dried thyme

- Salt and pepper to taste

Instructions:

1. Heat olive oil in a pot over medium heat. Add garlic and onion, sauté until translucent.

2. Add lentils, carrots, celery, thyme, salt, and pepper. Stir well.

3. Pour in vegetable broth, bring to a boil, then reduce heat and simmer for 30 minutes.

Nutritional Information (per serving):

- Calories: 280

- Protein: 16g

- Sodium: 220mg

- Potassium: 350mg

- Phosphorus: 200mg

10. Spinach and Feta Stuffed Chicken Breast

- **Prep Time:** 20 minutes

- **Cooking Time:** 30 minutes

- **Serving Size:** 1

Ingredients:

- 150g boneless, skinless chicken breast

- 1/4 cup fresh spinach leaves

- 1 tbsp crumbled feta cheese

- 1/2 tsp olive oil

- 1/2 tsp dried oregano

- Salt and pepper to taste

Instructions:

1. Preheat the oven to 375°F (190°C).

2. Cut a pocket into the chicken breast without cutting all the way through.

3. Stuff the pocket with fresh spinach leaves and feta cheese.

4. Rub the chicken with olive oil, dried oregano, salt, and pepper.

5. Bake for 25-30 minutes until the chicken is cooked through and juices run clear.

Nutritional Information (per serving):

- Calories: 240

- Protein: 30g

- Sodium: 220mg

- Potassium: 400mg

- Phosphorus: 180mg

DINNER RECIPES

1. Baked Lemon Herb Salmon

Prep Time: 10 minutes

Cooking Time: 20 minutes

Serving Size: 1

Ingredients:

- 150g salmon fillet

- 1 tablespoon fresh lemon juice

- 1 teaspoon olive oil

- 1/2 teaspoon dried thyme

- 1/2 teaspoon dried rosemary

- Pepper and salt

Instructions:

1. Preheat your oven to 375°F (190°C).

2. Place the salmon fillet on a baking sheet lined with parchment paper.

3. In a small bowl, mix the lemon juice, olive oil, thyme, rosemary, salt, and pepper.

4. Drizzle the mixture over the salmon.

5. Bake for approximately 20 minutes or until the salmon flakes easily with a fork.

6. Serve hot.

Nutritional Information (per serving):

- Calories: 220

- Protein: 28g

- Sodium: 80mg

- Potassium: 320mg

- Phosphorus: 180mg

2. Quinoa and Vegetable Stir-Fry

Prep Time: 15 minutes

Cooking Time: 20 minutes

Serving Size: 1

Ingredients:

- 1/2 cup cooked quinoa

- 1/2 cup broccoli florets

- 1/2 cup sliced bell peppers (red, yellow, or green)

- 1/2 cup sliced zucchini

- 1 tablespoon low-sodium soy sauce

- 1 teaspoon olive oil

- 1/2 teaspoon minced ginger

- 1/2 teaspoon minced garlic

- Pepper and salt

Instructions:

1. In a large skillet, heat olive oil over medium-high heat.

2. Add ginger and garlic, sauté for a minute.

3. Add broccoli, bell peppers, and zucchini. Stir-fry until tender.

4. Stir in cooked quinoa and soy sauce. Cook for an additional 2-3 minutes.

5. Season with pepper and salt.

6. Serve hot.

Nutritional Information (per serving):

- Calories: 290

- Protein: 9g

- Sodium: 270mg

- Potassium: 350mg

- Phosphorus: 110mg

3. Grilled Chicken with Asparagus

Prep Time: 15 minutes

Cooking Time: 15 minutes

Serving Size: 1

Ingredients:

- 150g skinless chicken breast

- 1/2 cup asparagus spears

- 1 teaspoon olive oil

- 1/2 teaspoon dried oregano

- 1/2 teaspoon garlic powder

- Pepper and salt

Instructions:

1. Preheat your grill to medium-high heat.

2. Brush the chicken breast and asparagus with olive oil.

3. Season the chicken with oregano, garlic powder, salt, and pepper.

4. Grill the chicken for about 6-7 minutes per side until cooked through.

5. Grill the asparagus until tender, about 5 minutes.

6. Serve hot.

Nutritional Information (per serving):

- Calories: 220

- Protein: 30g

- Sodium: 120mg

- Potassium: 380mg

- Phosphorus: 200mg

4. Lentil and Vegetable Soup

Prep Time: 15 minutes

Cooking Time: 45 minutes

Serving Size: 1

Ingredients:

- 1/2 cup dried green lentils

- 1/2 cup chopped carrots

- 1/2 cup chopped celery

- 1/2 cup chopped onion

- 1 clove garlic, minced

- 4 cups low-sodium vegetable broth

- 1/2 teaspoon dried thyme

- 1/2 teaspoon dried parsley

- Pepper and salt

Instructions:

1. In a large pot, sauté the onions and garlic in a little olive oil until fragrant.

2. Add carrots and celery, and cook for 5 minutes.

3. Stir in lentils, vegetable broth, thyme, parsley, salt, and pepper.

4. Bring to a boil, then reduce heat and simmer for about 40 minutes or until lentils are tender.

5. Serve hot.

Nutritional Information (per serving):

- Calories: 220

- Protein: 13g

- Sodium: 150mg

- Potassium: 580mg

- Phosphorus: 230mg

5. Turkey and Vegetable Skewers

Prep Time: 20 minutes

Cooking Time: 15 minutes

Serving Size: 1

Ingredients:

- 150g turkey breast, cut into cubes

- 1/2 cup bell peppers (red, yellow, or green), cut into chunks

- 1/2 cup zucchini, sliced

- 1/2 cup cherry tomatoes

- 1 teaspoon olive oil

- 1/2 teaspoon dried basil

- 1/2 teaspoon dried oregano

- Pepper and salt

Instructions:

1. Set your grill's temperature to medium-high.

2. Thread the turkey cubes, bell peppers, zucchini, and cherry tomatoes onto skewers.

3. Season the skewers with salt, pepper, basil, and oregano after brushing them with olive oil.

4. Grill for about 7-8 minutes per side, or until the turkey is cooked through.

5. Serve hot.

Nutritional Information (per serving):

- Calories: 230

- Protein: 28g

- Sodium: 90mg

- Potassium: 420mg

- Phosphorus: 190mg

6. Eggplant and Tomato Bake

Prep Time: 15 minutes

Cooking Time: 45 minutes

Serving Size: 1

Ingredients:

- 1 small eggplant, sliced

- 1 cup diced tomatoes (canned or fresh)

- 1/2 cup low-fat mozzarella cheese, shredded

- 1/2 teaspoon dried basil

- 1/2 teaspoon dried oregano

- Pepper and salt

Instructions:

1. Turn the oven on to 375°F, or 190°C.

2. In a baking dish, layer the sliced eggplant and diced tomatoes.

3. Sprinkle with basil, oregano, salt, and pepper.

4. Top with shredded mozzarella cheese.

5. Bake for approximately 40-45 minutes or until the eggplant is tender and the cheese is golden brown.

6. Serve hot.

Nutritional Information (per serving):

- Calories: 190

- Protein: 10g

- Sodium: 240mg

- Potassium: 580mg

- Phosphorus: 150mg

7. Lemon Garlic Shrimp Pasta

Prep Time: 10 minutes

Cooking Time: 20 minutes

Serving Size: 1

Ingredients:

- 150g whole wheat pasta

- 100g shrimp, peeled and deveined

- 1 tablespoon olive oil

- 1 clove garlic, minced

- Zest and juice of 1 lemon

- 1/2 teaspoon dried parsley

- Pepper and salt

Instructions:

1. Cook the whole wheat pasta according to package Instructions, then drain and set aside.

2. In a skillet, heat olive oil over medium heat.

3. Add minced garlic and sauté for about 1 minute.

4. Add shrimp and cook until pink and opaque, about 2-3 minutes per side.

5. Stir in lemon zest, lemon juice, dried parsley, salt, and pepper.

6. Toss the cooked pasta with the shrimp mixture.

7. Serve hot.

Nutritional Information (per serving):

- Calories: 320

- Protein: 20g

- Sodium: 150mg

- Potassium: 250mg

- Phosphorus: 200mg

8. Roasted Vegetable and Chickpea Salad

Prep Time: 15 minutes

Cooking Time: 25 minutes

Serving Size: 1

Ingredients:

- 1/2 cup chickpeas (canned or cooked)

- 1/2 cup mixed roasted vegetables (bell peppers, zucchini, cherry tomatoes)

- 1 tablespoon olive oil

- 1/2 teaspoon dried thyme

- 1/2 teaspoon paprika

- Pepper and salt

- 2 cups mixed greens

Instructions:

1. Set oven temperature to 400°F, or 200°C.

2. Toss the chickpeas and roasted vegetables with olive oil, thyme, paprika, salt, and pepper.

3. Roast in the oven for about 20-25 minutes or until vegetables are tender.

4. Serve the roasted mixture over a bed of mixed greens.

5. Drizzle with a light vinaigrette dressing if desired.

6. Serve warm or at room temperature.

Nutritional Information (per serving):

- Calories: 280

- Protein: 9g

- Sodium: 220mg

- Potassium: 350mg

- Phosphorus: 130mg

9. Turkey and Spinach Stuffed Bell Peppers

Prep Time: 20 minutes

Cooking Time: 40 minutes

Serving Size: 1 stuffed pepper

Ingredients:

- 1 bell pepper, halved and seeded

- 150g ground turkey (low fat)

- 1/2 cup chopped spinach

- 1/4 cup cooked brown rice

- 1/4 cup low-sodium tomato sauce

- 1/2 teaspoon dried Italian seasoning

- Pepper and salt

Instructions:

1. Preheat your oven to 350°F (175°C).

2. In a skillet, brown the ground turkey over medium heat. Drain any excess fat.

3. Stir in chopped spinach, cooked brown rice, tomato sauce, Italian seasoning, salt, and pepper.

4. Fill the bell pepper halves with the turkey mixture.

5. Place them in a baking dish and cover with foil.

6. Bake for about 30-40 minutes or until the peppers are tender.

7. Serve hot.

Nutritional Information (per serving - 1 stuffed pepper):

- Calories: 250

- Protein: 23g

- Sodium: 280mg

- Potassium: 350mg

- Phosphorus: 200mg

10. Sweet Potato and Black Bean Tacos

Prep Time: 15 minutes

Cooking Time: 25 minutes

Serving Size: 2 tacos

Ingredients:

- 2 small whole wheat tortillas

- 1 medium sweet potato, peeled and cubed

- 1/2 cup canned black beans, drained and rinsed

- 1/2 cup diced tomatoes (canned or fresh)

- 1/4 cup diced red onion

- 1/2 teaspoon chili powder

- 1/2 teaspoon ground cumin

- Pepper and salt

- Fresh cilantro leaves for garnish (optional)

Instructions:

1. Turn the oven on to 375°F, or 190°C.

2. Toss sweet potato cubes with olive oil, chili powder, cumin, salt, and pepper.

3. Roast in the oven for about 20-25 minutes or until the sweet potatoes are tender.

4. In a small saucepan, heat the black beans over low heat until warmed.

5. Warm the whole wheat tortillas in a dry skillet or microwave.

6. To assemble tacos, place a spoonful of roasted sweet potatoes in each tortilla, followed by black beans, diced tomatoes, and red onion.

7. Garnish with fresh cilantro leaves if desired.

8. Serve warm.

Nutritional Information (per serving - 2 tacos):

- Calories: 320

- Protein: 10g

- Sodium: 260mg

- Potassium: 600mg

- Phosphorus: 150mg

SNACKS AND DESSERTS RECIPES

1. Berry Parfait

Prep Time: 15 minutes

Cooking Time: 0 minutes

Serving Size: 1

Ingredients:

- 1/2 cup low-fat Greek yogurt

- 1/4 cup fresh mixed berries (strawberries, blueberries, raspberries)

- 1 tablespoon honey

- 1/4 cup low-phosphorus granola

Instructions:

1. Arrange the yogurt, mixed berries, and honey in a glass or bowl.

2. Top with a sprinkle of low-phosphorus granola.

3. Repeat the layers if desired.

4. Serve immediately or refrigerate for later.

Nutritional Information (per serving):

- Calories: 250

- Protein: 10g

- Sodium: 75mg

- Potassium: 200mg

- Phosphorus: 100mg

2. Cucumber and Hummus Snack

Prep Time: 10 minutes

Cooking Time: 0 minutes

Serving Size: 1

Ingredients:

- 1 medium cucumber, sliced

- 2 tablespoons low-sodium hummus

- A pinch of fresh dill (optional)

Instructions:

1. Arrange the cucumber slices on a plate.

2. Serve with a side of low-sodium hummus for dipping.

3. Garnish with fresh dill if desired.

Nutritional Information (per serving):

- Calories: 100

- Protein: 4g

- Sodium: 50mg

- Potassium: 150mg

- Phosphorus: 40mg

3. Baked Apple with Cinnamon

Prep Time: 10 minutes

Cooking Time: 20 minutes

Serving Size: 1

Ingredients:

- 1 medium apple, cored and sliced

- 1/2 teaspoon ground cinnamon

- 1 tablespoon honey (optional)

Instructions:

1. Preheat the oven to 350°F (175°C).

2. Place apple slices in a baking dish, sprinkle with cinnamon, and drizzle with honey if desired.

3. Bake for 20 minutes or until the apples are tender.

4. Serve warm.

Nutritional Information (per serving):

- Calories: 100

- Protein: 0g

- Sodium: 0mg

- Potassium: 150mg

- Phosphorus: 10mg

4. Guacamole and Carrot Sticks

Prep Time: 15 minutes

Cooking Time: 0 minutes

Serving Size: 1

Ingredients:

- 1 small avocado, mashed

- 1/4 teaspoon garlic powder

- 1/4 teaspoon onion powder

- 1 small carrot, sliced into sticks

- Lime juice (optional)

Instructions:

1. In a bowl, mix mashed avocado with garlic and onion powder.

2. Serve with carrot sticks for dipping.

3. Squeeze lime juice over the guacamole if desired.

Nutritional Information (per serving):

- Calories: 200

- Protein: 2g

- Sodium: 20mg

- Potassium: 400mg

- Phosphorus: 50mg

5. Frozen Banana Pops

Prep Time: 10 minutes

Freezing Time: 2 hours

Serving Size: 1

Ingredients:

- 1 ripe banana, peeled and cut in half

- 2 tablespoons low-fat yogurt (plain or flavored)

- 1 tablespoon chopped nuts (e.g., almonds or walnuts)

Instructions:

1. Insert Popsicle sticks into the cut ends of the banana halves.

2. Dip the bananas into the yogurt, coating them evenly.

3. Roll the yogurt-covered banana in chopped nuts.

4. Place on a parchment paper-lined tray and freeze for at least 2 hours.

Nutritional Information (per serving):

- Calories: 150

- Protein: 3g

- Sodium: 20mg

- Potassium: 350mg

- Phosphorus: 40mg

6. Tuna Salad Lettuce Wraps

Prep Time: 15 minutes

Cooking Time: 0 minutes

Serving Size: 1

Ingredients:

- 1 can (5 oz.) low-sodium tuna, drained

- 2 tablespoons low-fat mayonnaise

- 1/4 cup finely chopped celery

- 1/4 cup diced red bell pepper

- 2 large lettuce leaves (such as iceberg or Romaine)

Instructions:

1. In a bowl, mix tuna, low-fat mayonnaise, celery, and red bell pepper.

2. Spoon the tuna salad mixture onto lettuce leaves.

3. Roll the lettuce leaves to form wraps.

4. Serve immediately.

Nutritional Information (per serving):

- Calories: 250

- Protein: 25g

- Sodium: 150mg

- Potassium: 300mg

- Phosphorus: 150mg

7. Cottage Cheese with Pineapple

Prep Time: 5 minutes

Cooking Time: 0 minutes

Serving Size: 1

Ingredients:

- 1/2 cup low-fat cottage cheese

- 1/4 cup canned pineapple chunks (in juice, drained)

- A sprinkle of cinnamon (optional)

Instructions:

1. In a bowl, combine cottage cheese and pineapple chunks.

2. Sprinkle with a pinch of cinnamon if desired.

3. Serve chilled.

Nutritional Information (per serving):

- Calories: 150

- Protein: 14g

- Sodium: 300mg

- Potassium: 180mg

- Phosphorus: 100mg

8. Quinoa and Fruit Salad

Prep Time: 20 minutes

Cooking Time: 15 minutes

Serving Size: 1

Ingredients:

- 1/2 cup cooked quinoa

- 1/4 cup diced fresh fruit (e.g., berries, apples, or pears)

- 1 tablespoon chopped mint leaves

- 1 tablespoon honey (optional)

Instructions:

1. In a bowl, combine cooked quinoa and diced fruit.

2. Add chopped mint leaves and drizzle with honey if desired.

3. Toss gently to mix.

4. Serve as a refreshing salad.

Nutritional Information (per serving):

- Calories: 200

- Protein: 5g

- Sodium: 10mg

- Potassium: 200mg

- Phosphorus: 80mg

9. Banana and Almond Butter Toast

Prep Time: 5 minutes

Cooking Time: 5 minutes

Serving Size: 1

Ingredients:

- 1 slice whole-grain bread (low-phosphorus)

- 1 tablespoon almond butter

- 1/2 banana, sliced

Instructions:

1. Toast the whole-grain bread.

2. Spread almond butter on the toast.

3. Top with banana slices.

4. Enjoy as an easy and healthy snack.

Nutritional Information (per serving):

- Calories: 250

- Protein: 7g

- Sodium: 150mg

- Potassium: 250mg

- Phosphorus: 100mg

10. Chia Seed Pudding

Prep Time: 5 minutes (plus chilling time)

Cooking Time: 0 minutes

Serving Size: 1

Ingredients:

- 2 tablespoons chia seeds

- 1/2 cup unsweetened almond milk

- 1/4 teaspoon vanilla extract

- 1 tablespoon sliced strawberries (optional)

Instructions:

1. In a jar, combine chia seeds, almond milk, and vanilla extract.

2. Stir well, ensuring the chia seeds are fully immersed in the liquid.

3. Put it in the fridge to thicken for at least two hours, or overnight.

4. Top with sliced strawberries before serving if desired.

Nutritional Information (per serving):

- Calories: 150

- Protein: 5g

- Sodium: 80mg

- Potassium: 120mg

- Phosphorus: 80mg

BEVERAGES AND DRINKS

1. Refreshing Watermelon Cooler

Prep Time: 10 minutes

Cooking Time: 0 minutes

Serving Size: 1

Ingredients:

- 1 cup fresh watermelon, diced

- 1/2 cup ice cubes

- 1 tablespoon fresh lime juice

- 1 teaspoon honey (optional)

- Fresh mint leaves for garnish

Instructions:

1. Place the diced watermelon and ice cubes in a blender.

2. Add fresh lime juice and honey (if desired).

3. Blend until smooth.

4. Pour into a glass, garnish with fresh mint leaves, and serve.

Nutritional Information (per serving):

- Calories: 60

- Protein: 1g

- Sodium: 2mg

- Potassium: 150mg

- Phosphorus: 10mg

2. Cranberry Apple Iced Tea

Prep Time: 5 minutes

Cooking Time: 5 minutes

Serving Size: 1

Ingredients:

- 1 cup unsweetened cranberry juice

- 1 cup unsweetened apple juice

- 1 black tea bag

- 1 cup boiling water

- Ice cubes

- Fresh apple slices for garnish

Instructions:

1. Steep the black tea bag in boiling water for 3-5 minutes; let it cool.

2. In a pitcher, combine the cranberry juice, apple juice, and cooled tea.

3. Add ice cubes and stir.

4. Garnish with fresh apple slices and serve.

Nutritional Information (per serving):

- Calories: 80

- Protein: 0.5g

- Sodium: 5mg

- Potassium: 100mg

- Phosphorus: 10mg

3. Cucumber and Mint Infused Water

Prep Time: 5 minutes

Cooking Time: 0 minutes

Serving Size: 1

Ingredients:

- 1/2 cucumber, sliced

- 5-6 fresh mint leaves

- 1 cup ice cubes

- 1 cup water

Instructions:

1. Place cucumber slices and fresh mint leaves in a glass or pitcher.

2. Add ice cubes.

3. Pour water over the ingredients.

4. Let it infuse for a few minutes before serving.

Nutritional Information (per serving):

- Calories: 0

- Protein: 0g

- Sodium: 0mg

- Potassium: 50mg

- Phosphorus: 0mg

4. Berry Blast Smoothie

Prep Time: 5 minutes

Cooking Time: 0 minutes

Serving Size: 1

Ingredients:

- 1/2 cup mixed berries (blueberries, strawberries, raspberries)

- 1/2 banana

- 1/2 cup plain Greek yogurt (low-fat)

- 1/2 cup unsweetened almond milk

- 1 tablespoon honey (optional)

Instructions:

1. Place mixed berries, banana, Greek yogurt, almond milk, and honey (if desired) in a blender.

2. Blend until smooth.

3. Pour into a glass and serve immediately.

Nutritional Information (per serving):

- Calories: 200

- Protein: 11g

- Sodium: 80mg

- Potassium: 350mg

- Phosphorus: 150mg

5. Green Vegetable Juice

Prep Time: 10 minutes

Cooking Time: 0 minutes

Serving Size: 1

Ingredients:

- 1 cup spinach leaves

- 1/2 cucumber

- 1 celery stalk

- 1/2 green apple

- 1/2 lemon, peeled

- 1/2 cup water

Instructions:

1. Wash and chop the vegetables and apple.

2. Place them in a juicer or blender with water.

3. Blend until smooth and strain if needed.

4. Pour into a glass and serve chilled.

Nutritional Information (per serving):

- Calories: 50

- Protein: 1.5g

- Sodium: 50mg

- Potassium: 350mg

- Phosphorus: 30mg

6. Creamy Avocado Smoothie

Prep Time: 5 minutes

Cooking Time: 0 minutes

Serving Size: 1

Ingredients:

- 1/2 ripe avocado

- 1/2 cup plain Greek yogurt (low-fat)

- 1/2 cup unsweetened almond milk

- 1 tablespoon honey (optional)

- 1/2 teaspoon vanilla extract

- Ice cubes (optional)

Instructions:

1. Scoop out the ripe avocado and place it in a blender.

2. Add Greek yogurt, almond milk, honey (if desired), and vanilla extract.

3. Blend until creamy.

4. Add ice cubes if you prefer a colder smoothie.

5. Pour into a glass and serve.

Nutritional Information (per serving):

- Calories: 200

- Protein: 10g

- Sodium: 90mg

- Potassium: 420mg

- Phosphorus: 110mg

7. Lemon-Parsley Detox Water

Prep Time: 5 minutes

Cooking Time: 0 minutes

Serving Size: 1

Ingredients:

- 1 lemon, thinly sliced

- Fresh parsley leaves

- 1 cup ice cubes

- 1 cup water

Instructions:

1. Place lemon slices and fresh parsley leaves in a glass or pitcher.

2. Add ice cubes.

3. Pour water over the ingredients.

4. Allow it to infuse for a few minutes before serving.

Nutritional Information (per serving):

- Calories: 0

- Protein: 0g

- Sodium: 0mg

- Potassium: 50mg

- Phosphorus: 0mg

8. Ginger and Turmeric Tea

Prep Time: 5 minutes

Cooking Time: 10 minutes

Serving Size: 1

Ingredients:

- 1 cup water

- 1/2 teaspoon grated ginger

- 1/2 teaspoon ground turmeric

- 1 teaspoon honey (optional)

- A slice of lemon (for garnish)

Instructions:

1. In a small saucepan, bring water to a boil.

2. Add grated ginger and ground turmeric, then reduce heat and simmer for 10 minutes.

3. Strain the tea into a cup, and add honey if desired.

4. Garnish with a slice of lemon.

Nutritional Information (per serving):

- Calories: 10

- Protein: 0g

- Sodium: 0mg

- Potassium: 20mg

- Phosphorus: 0mg

9. Blueberry-Pomegranate Smoothie

Prep Time: 5 minutes

Cooking Time: 0 minutes

Serving Size: 1

Ingredients:

- 1/2 cup frozen blueberries

- 1/4 cup pomegranate seeds

- 1/2 cup plain Greek yogurt (low-fat)

- 1/2 cup unsweetened almond milk

- 1 tablespoon honey (optional)

Instructions:

1. Place frozen blueberries, pomegranate seeds, Greek yogurt, almond milk, and honey (if desired) in a blender.

2. Blend until smooth.

3. Pour into a glass and serve immediately.

Nutritional Information (per serving):

- Calories: 180

- Protein: 10g

- Sodium: 80mg

- Potassium: 240mg

- Phosphorus: 120mg

10. Minty Green Tea Cooler

Prep Time: 10 minutes

Cooking Time: 0 minutes

Serving Size: 1

Ingredients:

- 1 green tea bag

- 1 cup boiling water

- 4-5 fresh mint leaves

- 1/2 teaspoon honey (optional)

- Ice cubes

Instructions:

1. Steep the green tea bag in boiling water for 3-5 minutes; let it cool.

2. Add fresh mint leaves and honey (if desired).

3. Stir well and chill in the refrigerator.

4. Serve over ice cubes.

Nutritional Information (per serving):

- Calories: 5

- Protein: 0g

- Sodium: 5mg

- Potassium: 10mg

- Phosphorus: 0mg

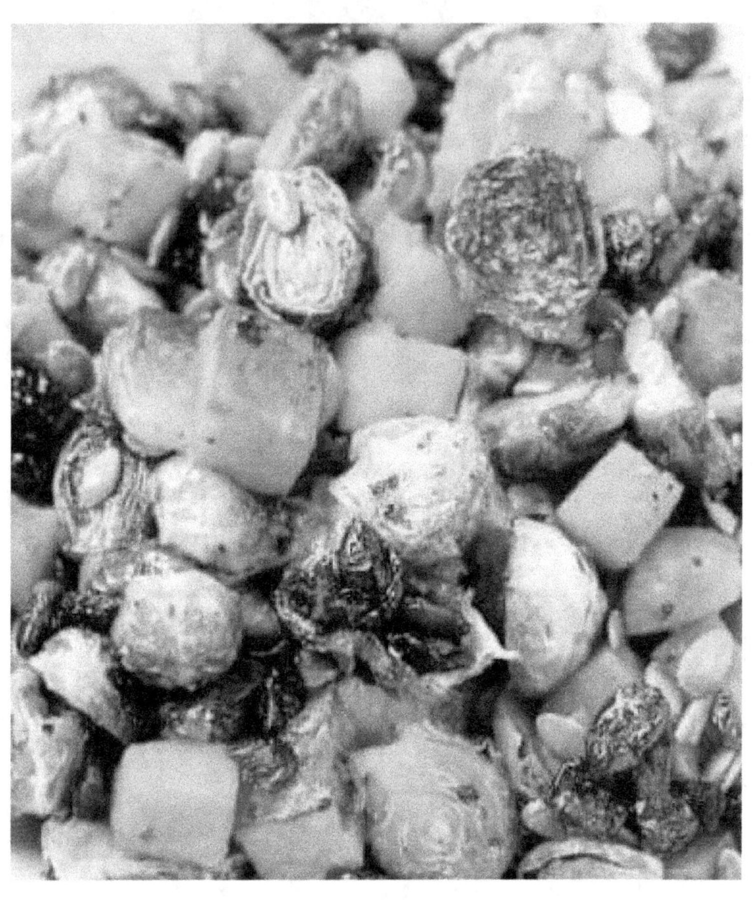

CHAPTER 3

30 DAYS MEAL PLAN

Day 1:
- Breakfast: Creamy Oatmeal with Berries
- Lunch: Creamy Chicken and Vegetable Soup
- Dinner: Baked Lemon Herb Salmon
- Snack: Berry Parfait

Day 2:
- Breakfast: Scrambled Egg Whites with Spinach
- Lunch: Lemon Garlic Shrimp and Asparagus
- Dinner: Quinoa and Vegetable Stir-Fry
- Snack: Cucumber and Hummus Snack

Day 3:
- Breakfast: Banana Almond Smoothie
- Lunch: Quinoa and Vegetable Stir-Fry
- Dinner: Grilled Chicken with Asparagus
- Snack: Baked Apple with Cinnamon

Day 4:
- Breakfast: Greek Yogurt Parfait with Nuts and Berries
- Lunch: Salmon and Spinach Salad
- Dinner: Lentil and Vegetable Soup
- Snack: Guacamole and Carrot Sticks

Day 5:
- Breakfast: Spinach and Mushroom Breakfast Quesadilla
- Lunch: Mushroom and Spinach Omelette
- Dinner: Turkey and Vegetable Skewers
- Snack: Frozen Banana Pops

Day 6:
- Breakfast: Quinoa Breakfast Bowl
- Lunch: Grilled Lemon Herb Chicken Salad
- Dinner: Eggplant and Tomato Bake
- Snack: Tuna Salad Lettuce Wraps

Day 7:
- Breakfast: Sweet Potato Hash with Eggs
- Lunch: Black Bean and Vegetable Tacos
- Dinner: Lemon Garlic Shrimp Pasta
- Snack: Cottage Cheese with Pineapple

Day 8:
- Breakfast: Blueberry Cottage Cheese Pancakes
- Lunch: Baked Lemon Garlic Tilapia
- Dinner: Roasted Vegetable and Chickpea Salad
- Snack: Quinoa and Fruit Salad

Day 9:
- Breakfast: Avocado and Tomato Toast
- Lunch: Vegetable and Lentil Soup
- Dinner: Turkey and Spinach Stuffed Bell Peppers

- Snack: Banana and Almond Butter Toast

Day 10:
- Breakfast: Chia Seed Pudding
- Lunch: Spinach and Feta Stuffed Chicken Breast
- Dinner: Sweet Potato and Black Bean Tacos
- Snack: Chia Seed Pudding

Day 11:
- Breakfast: Creamy Oatmeal with Berries
- Lunch: Creamy Chicken and Vegetable Soup
- Dinner: Baked Lemon Herb Salmon
- Snack: Berry Parfait

Day 12:
- Breakfast: Scrambled Egg Whites with Spinach
- Lunch: Lemon Garlic Shrimp and Asparagus
- Dinner: Quinoa and Vegetable Stir-Fry
- Snack: Cucumber and Hummus Snack

Day 13:
- Breakfast: Banana Almond Smoothie
- Lunch: Quinoa and Vegetable Stir-Fry
- Dinner: Grilled Chicken with Asparagus
- Snack: Baked Apple with Cinnamon

Day 14:
- Breakfast: Greek Yogurt Parfait with Nuts and Berries
- Lunch: Salmon and Spinach Salad
- Dinner: Lentil and Vegetable Soup
- Snack: Guacamole and Carrot Sticks

Day 15:
- Breakfast: Spinach and Mushroom Breakfast Quesadilla
- Lunch: Mushroom and Spinach Omelette
- Dinner: Turkey and Vegetable Skewers
- Snack: Frozen Banana Pops

Day 16:
- Breakfast: Quinoa Breakfast Bowl
- Lunch: Grilled Lemon Herb Chicken Salad
- Dinner: Eggplant and Tomato Bake
- Snack: Tuna Salad Lettuce Wraps

Day 17:
- Breakfast: Sweet Potato Hash with Eggs
- Lunch: Black Bean and Vegetable Tacos
- Dinner: Lemon Garlic Shrimp Pasta
- Snack: Cottage Cheese with Pineapple

Day 18:
- Breakfast: Blueberry Cottage Cheese Pancakes
- Lunch: Baked Lemon Garlic Tilapia
- Dinner: Roasted Vegetable and Chickpea Salad
- Snack: Quinoa and Fruit Salad

Day 19:
- Breakfast: Avocado and Tomato Toast
- Lunch: Vegetable and Lentil Soup
- Dinner: Turkey and Spinach Stuffed Bell Peppers
- Snack: Banana and Almond Butter Toast

Day 20:
- Breakfast: Chia Seed Pudding
- Lunch: Spinach and Feta Stuffed Chicken Breast
- Dinner: Sweet Potato and Black Bean Tacos
- Snack: Chia Seed Pudding

Day 21:
- Breakfast: Creamy Oatmeal with Berries
- Lunch: Creamy Chicken and Vegetable Soup
- Dinner: Baked Lemon Herb Salmon
- Snack: Berry Parfait

Day 22:
- Breakfast: Scrambled Egg Whites with Spinach
- Lunch: Lemon Garlic Shrimp and Asparagus
- Dinner: Quinoa and Vegetable Stir-Fry
- Snack: Cucumber and Hummus Snack

Day 23:
- Breakfast: Banana Almond Smoothie
- Lunch: Quinoa and Vegetable Stir-Fry
- Dinner: Grilled Chicken with Asparagus

- Snack: Baked Apple with Cinnamon

Day 24:
- Breakfast: Greek Yogurt Parfait with Nuts and Berries
- Lunch: Salmon and Spinach Salad
- Dinner: Lentil and Vegetable Soup
- Snack: Guacamole and Carrot Sticks

Day 25:
- Breakfast: Spinach and Mushroom Breakfast Quesadilla
- Lunch: Mushroom and Spinach Omelette
- Dinner: Turkey and Vegetable Skewers
- Snack: Frozen Banana Pops

Day 26:
- Breakfast: Quinoa Breakfast Bowl
- Lunch: Grilled Lemon Herb Chicken Salad
- Dinner: Eggplant and Tomato Bake
- Snack: Tuna Salad Lettuce Wraps

Day 27:
- Breakfast: Sweet Potato Hash with Eggs
- Lunch: Black Bean and Vegetable Tacos
- Dinner: Lemon Garlic Shrimp Pasta
- Snack: Cottage Cheese with Pineapple

Day 28:
- Breakfast: Blueberry Cottage Cheese Pancakes
- Lunch: Baked Lemon Garlic Tilapia
- Dinner: Roasted Vegetable and Chickpea Salad
- Snack: Quinoa and Fruit Salad

Day 29:
- Breakfast: Avocado and Tomato Toast
- Lunch: Vegetable and Lentil Soup
- Dinner: Turkey and Spinach Stuffed Bell Peppers
- Snack: Banana and Almond Butter Toast

Day 30:
- Breakfast: Chia Seed Pudding
- Lunch: Spinach and Feta Stuffed Chicken Breast
- Dinner: Sweet Potato and Black Bean Tacos
- Snack: Chia Seed Pudding

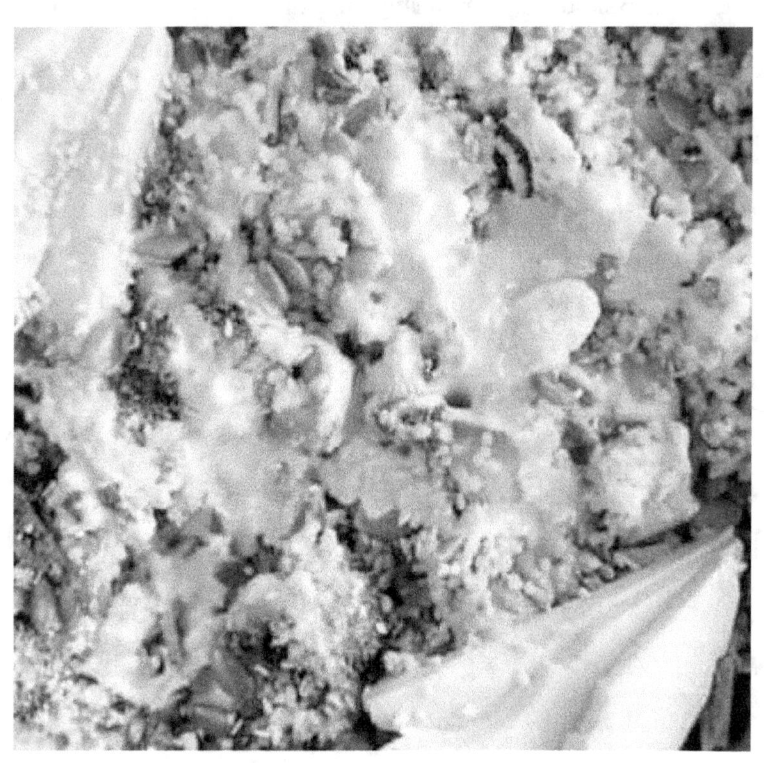

CONCLUSION

As we reach the end of "Kidney Disease Diet Cookbook for Women," it's essential to reflect on the journey you've embarked upon. This cookbook has been more than just a collection of recipes; it's a guide, a companion, and a source of inspiration for women navigating the complexities of kidney disease through the power of nutrition.

Each recipe was crafted with the utmost care, keeping in mind the unique dietary needs of women with kidney disease. From breakfasts to dinners, snacks to beverages, every dish was designed to nourish your body while delighting your palate. The ingredients chosen were not just for their kidney-friendly properties, but also for their ability to foster overall health and well-being.

But "Kidney Disease Diet Cookbook for Women," is more than a compilation of recipes. It's a testament to the resilience and strength that lies within each one of you. It recognizes the challenges you face and offers a way to take control of your health and your life through informed, delicious dietary choices.

As you continue on your path, remember that your diet is a powerful tool in managing kidney disease. Each meal is an opportunity to nourish your body and support your kidneys. With "Kidney Disease Diet Cookbook for Women," you have the resources to make each bite count.

And finally, a word of motivation: You are not alone on this journey. Every step you take towards better health is a victory, every healthy meal an achievement. You have the power to make positive changes, and this cookbook is here to guide you along the way. Embrace the journey with confidence and optimism, knowing that you're doing something wonderful for your body and your spirit.

Here's to your health, to your strength, and to a future filled with flavorful, kidney-friendly meals. Keep nourishing, keep healing, and keep thriving!

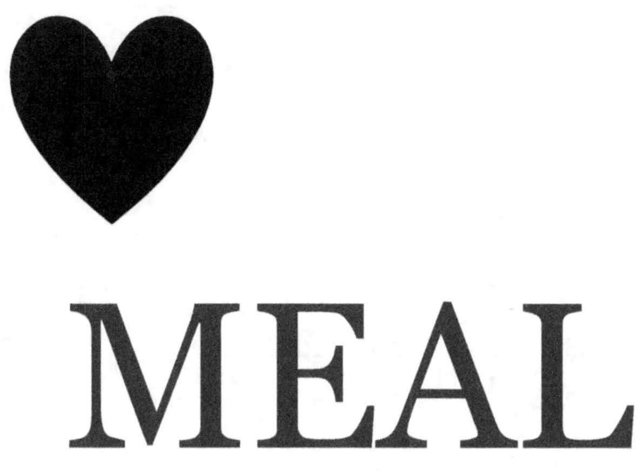

MEAL PLANNER

Monday	Breakfast	Lunch	Dinner

Tuesday	Breakfast	Lunch	Dinner

Wednesday	Breakfast	Lunch	Dinner

Thursday	Breakfast	Lunch	Dinner

Friday	Breakfast	Lunch	Dinner

Saturday	Breakfast	Lunch	Dinner

Sunday	Breakfast	Lunch	Dinner

Monday	Breakfast	Lunch	Dinner

Tuesday	Breakfast	Lunch	Dinner

Wednesday	Breakfast	Lunch	Dinner

Thursday	Breakfast	Lunch	Dinner

Friday	Breakfast	Lunch	Dinner

Saturday	Breakfast	Lunch	Dinner

Sunday	Breakfast	Lunch	Dinner

Monday	Breakfast	Lunch	Dinner

Tuesday	Breakfast	Lunch	Dinner

Wednesday	Breakfast	Lunch	Dinner

Thursday	Breakfast	Lunch	Dinner

Friday	Breakfast	Lunch	Dinner

Saturday	Breakfast	Lunch	Dinner

Sunday	Breakfast	Lunch	Dinner

Monday	Breakfast	Lunch	Dinner

Tuesday	Breakfast	Lunch	Dinner

Wednesday	Breakfast	Lunch	Dinner

Thursday	Breakfast	Lunch	Dinner

Friday	Breakfast	Lunch	Dinner

Saturday	Breakfast	Lunch	Dinner

Sunday	Breakfast	Lunch	Dinner

Monday	Breakfast	Lunch	Dinner

Tuesday	Breakfast	Lunch	Dinner

Wednesday	Breakfast	Lunch	Dinner

Thursday	Breakfast	Lunch	Dinner

Friday	Breakfast	Lunch	Dinner

Saturday	Breakfast	Lunch	Dinner

Sunday	Breakfast	Lunch	Dinner

Monday	Breakfast	Lunch	Dinner

Tuesday	Breakfast	Lunch	Dinner

Wednesday	Breakfast	Lunch	Dinner

Thursday	Breakfast	Lunch	Dinner

Friday	Breakfast	Lunch	Dinner

Saturday	Breakfast	Lunch	Dinner

Sunday	Breakfast	Lunch	Dinner

Monday	Breakfast	Lunch	Dinner

Tuesday	Breakfast	Lunch	Dinner

Wednesday	Breakfast	Lunch	Dinner

Thursday	Breakfast	Lunch	Dinner

Friday	Breakfast	Lunch	Dinner

Saturday	Breakfast	Lunch	Dinner

Sunday	Breakfast	Lunch	Dinner

Monday	Breakfast	Lunch	Dinner

Tuesday	Breakfast	Lunch	Dinner

Wednesday	Breakfast	Lunch	Dinner

Thursday	Breakfast	Lunch	Dinner

Friday	Breakfast	Lunch	Dinner

Saturday	Breakfast	Lunch	Dinner

Sunday	Breakfast	Lunch	Dinner

Monday	Breakfast	Lunch	Dinner

Tuesday	Breakfast	Lunch	Dinner

Wednesday	Breakfast	Lunch	Dinner

Thursday	Breakfast	Lunch	Dinner

Friday	Breakfast	Lunch	Dinner

Saturday	Breakfast	Lunch	Dinner

Sunday	Breakfast	Lunch	Dinner

<table>
<tr><td rowspan="2">Monday</td><td>Breakfast</td><td>Lunch</td><td>Dinner</td></tr>
<tr><td></td><td></td><td></td></tr>
<tr><td rowspan="2">Tuesday</td><td>Breakfast</td><td>Lunch</td><td>Dinner</td></tr>
<tr><td></td><td></td><td></td></tr>
<tr><td rowspan="2">Wednesday</td><td>Breakfast</td><td>Lunch</td><td>Dinner</td></tr>
<tr><td></td><td></td><td></td></tr>
<tr><td rowspan="2">Thursday</td><td>Breakfast</td><td>Lunch</td><td>Dinner</td></tr>
<tr><td></td><td></td><td></td></tr>
<tr><td rowspan="2">Friday</td><td>Breakfast</td><td>Lunch</td><td>Dinner</td></tr>
<tr><td></td><td></td><td></td></tr>
<tr><td rowspan="2">Saturday</td><td>Breakfast</td><td>Lunch</td><td>Dinner</td></tr>
<tr><td></td><td></td><td></td></tr>
<tr><td rowspan="2">Sunday</td><td>Breakfast</td><td>Lunch</td><td>Dinner</td></tr>
<tr><td></td><td></td><td></td></tr>
</table>